G

OVERCOMING
FOOD ADDICTION:
HOW TO STOP
BINGE EATING

Health Research Staff

Published by:
Millwood Media
PO Box 1220
Melrose, FL 32666 USA

www.MillwoodMediaEpub.com

ISBN 13: 978-1-937918-69-9

Health Disclaimer:

Any and all information contained herein is not intended to take the place of medical advice from a healthcare professional. Any action taken based on these contents is at the sole discretion and liability of the reader.

Readers should always consult appropriate health professionals on any matter relating to their health and well-being before taking any action of any kind concerning health-related issues.

Any information or opinions provided here or in any Millwood Media related articles, materials or information are believed to be accurate and sound. However, Millwood Media assumes no liability for the use or misuse of information provided by Millwood Media.

No personnel or associates of Millwood Media will in any way be held responsible by any reader who fails to consult the appropriate health authorities with respect to their individual healthcare before acting on or using any information contained herein. And neither the author nor publisher of any of this information will be held responsible for errors or omissions, or use or misuse of the information.

Contents

Introduction 1

1. Physical Aspects 5

   • Remove Problem Foods 6

   • Grocery Shop for Healthier Alternatives 8

   • Never Shop Without a Grocery List 9

   • Avoid Intense Diets 10

   • Toss Take-Out Menus 11

   • Stay Busy 12

   • Eliminate Distractions 13

   • Eating Regularly Throughout the Day 14

   • Adopt a Healthy Exercise Program 16

   • Eating a Lower Carb Diet 17

   • Meditation and Yoga 19

   • Summary 20

2. Psychological Aspects 21

   • Positive Self-Statements 21

   • Strength Training 23

   • Recognizing Justifications 25

   • Toss Fashion and Fitness Magazines 26

   • Eliminating Feelings of Helplessness 28

3. Emotional Aspects **31**

   • Journaling 32

   • Counseling 33

   • Find Passion in Activities 34

   • Visualizing 37

   • Find Healthier Replacements 37

Now What? **41**

Bonus Book:
  Easy Weight Loss With EFT **49**

Introduction

In a world obsessed with dieting, and all the different weight loss tactics that go along with it, one very serious issue that often sneaks under the radar is binge eating.

A lot of people downplay binge eating as just 'loving food too much.' But it can be an extremely serious problem to the extent it causes them to gain more and more weight. Examined closer, you'll see it's very complex as it touches upon a number of different physical, mental, and emotional components.

Binge eating can be deeply rooted in behavior patterns, and for some people food is the mechanism they use to cope. Much like any addiction, food causes a chemical release in the body very much like drugs and alcohol, and provides a temporary escape from the difficulties of life for a short period of time. (Carbohydrates for example, cause a heavy hit of serotonin which induces feelings of calm and relaxation.)

When you're stressed and feel like you need something to calm you down, you may crave simple carbs (that break down into sugar). Should you give in and eat a big "dose" of them, you're going to get powerful relaxation and calming benefits. During your very first episode of binging, you learn the power food can have over how you feel. And once that realization is made, it can be a very hard connection to break.

Dealing with the reasons you binge eat can be more work than you're willing to put in, as it's far easier to self-medicate with food as an escape from your problems.

Many people don't understand the full ramifications of binge eating as they see it as an issue with maintaining a proper body weight. But it's far more than that as it places strain on the digestive and pulmonary system. Rapid rates of fat gain put you at risk for heart disease, high cholesterol and blood pressure, as well as diabetes.

If you starve yourself to prevent weight gain because you're binging too often and too much, you'll run the risk of many health problems. It's very likely you'll begin to experience nutritional deficiencies due to the fact you're replacing healthy food with much less healthy choices. Furthermore, this can also cause a sluggish metabolism, lean muscle mass loss, and even threaten the health of your bones due to lack of calcium and Vitamin D.

Binge eating causes a great deal of harm beyond weight gain. So it's critical you come to terms with your disorder (and yes, it is a disorder) so you can realize just how serious the situation is.

There's no denying the fact that human beings take pleasure in food. It's when they let the pleasure factor get out of control and start relying on eating to make them feel better rather than looking for pleasure from their everyday life that problems are more likely to develop.

Society makes it easy to binge. In any grocery store you're greeted with aisles of processed snack foods that contain highly refined carbs, fat, salt, or other ingredients your body is craving. In a world where you can super-size a fast food meal, and purchase chocolate bars and bags of chips in colossal sizes, it's far too easy to overeat unless you have a good handle on your choices and emotional drives.

This guide is going to discuss the main areas that contribute to binge eating, and give you some excellent techniques to help you overcome your problem.

Will it be easy? Of course not. There's no sense in minimizing the issue, because it will set you up for unrealistic expectations and disappointment. But as long as you stay committed to the goal to break free from emotional eating, it most definitely is possible.

It will get easier with each battle you win. Obviously the first few days will be the hardest. But with each step you take to become binge-free, the next will be a little bit easier. The longer you stay on task, the closer you'll get to being free from this condition forever and reaching your dream body, as well as improving your health and fitness goals.

If you're ready to take control of your life, let's begin by discussing the physical aspects of binge eating to help you put this problem behind you.

* * *

Attention All Eagle Eyes: We've had a number of people proof this book before we released it to you, but there is a chance you might spot something that was missed. If you find a typo or other obvious error please send it to us. And if you're the first one to report it, we'll send you a free gift! Send to: millwoodmedia@gmail.com

1. *Physical* ASPECTS

The physical aspects of binge eating refer to the elements that make a binge possible. If you want to reduce the chances of going on a binge and put a stop to this unfortunate condition, it's important to take control over your choices.

Dealing with the mental and emotional elements as they arise go a long way towards putting a stop to binge eating forever (and they must be addressed, or you'll encounter them again at some point in your life).

Taking control of the physical elements from the onset will make it difficult for you to go on another binge. Following are some tips you can implement to stop binge eating before it gets to that point.

Remove Problem Foods

The first thing you should do to kick-start your journey is to go through your cupboards and fridge and remove any food you tend to eat during a binge. This includes cookies, crackers, cereals, chips, chocolate bars, frozen novelties – basically anything in large quantities (grabbing handfuls of food is mindless eating and deadly to your diet).

One common myth people have is that binging is about eating as much 'junk food' as possible. They imagine someone shoving Oreos into their mouth with one hand, while holding a spoonful of cookie dough ice cream in the other.

But you can also binge on healthy food (whole grain bread for example) by helping yourself to ten slices of bread piled with peanut butter. While this kind of snack wouldn't normally be considered bad, eating that much indicates a red flag.

So you want to be thinking about which foods are triggers that make you want them in high quantities. Regardless of the nutritional information, if you feel you could eat more than you should it should be removed while you're getting your eating habits under control.

Most people aren't going to sit down and eat five chicken breasts or three bowls of broccoli. So for the most part you won't be removing healthy food you should have in your diet. But you will be removing unhealthy junk food in addition to considering potential threats masked as "healthy" (i.e., the whole grain bread and peanut butter above).

You need to talk to everyone you live with (friends, family, roommates), and ask them to avoid bringing problem food into the house. Or if they do, they'll need to hide them so you aren't aware they're there. Of course, this will involve opening up to others about your concerns, and different people will have different comfort levels about how to respond. But a good support system is key to overcoming any mental battle, whether it's binge eating, depression, or a drug addiction.

Try to keep in mind that everyone experiences a multitude of problems over their lifetime, and you're no different. People with binge eating issues tend to be very embarrassed about their condition. But it is a situation you can overcome and there's no reason to feel ashamed.

The important people in your life will offer you support as you work through the steps to overcome binge eating. (If they don't, you may want to question whether you want them your life in the first place.) But if you're brave enough to reach out and talk to them, you might surprise yourself at how understanding they are, and how willing they are to help you overcome your addiction.

Grocery Shop for Healthier Alternatives

Having problem foods in your kitchen will make them readily available for a binge. So the next thing on your list of physical elements to control is to learn how to grocery shop to prevent that from happening. If you stock healthy food that keeps you satisfied and your body well-fueled, you'll not only nourish your body but will be far less likely to binge.

While some people binge on healthy food just because any food will do, most people want high sugar, high fat food that brings them physical pleasure as this provides the greatest escape. That is after all what they're looking for.

Many people were given food as a reward when they were children. If they played nicely, they got a cookie. If they cleaned their room, they were given ice cream. Straight A's meant extra helpings at the dinner table. They weren't usually given oatmeal or brown rice when they did something good, so they can't view healthy foods as a way to make them feel better. And now as adults they associate joy and feeling good with food, which is what causes them to lean towards 'treat' foods and the ugly cycle continues.

Therefore, having healthy food available you see as fuel for your body rather than as a reward or panacea for your problems will help you cut ties with binge eating. You'll want to have proteins such as chicken and turkey breast, red meat, egg whites, fish, seafood, and low-fat dairy products stocked in your larder.

On the carbohydrate side turn to oatmeal, brown rice, quinoa, sweet potatoes, fresh fruits, and plenty of vegetables. Whole wheat bread and pasta are acceptable as long as they aren't problem food for you (do a deep assessment of your behavior and cravings to discover if they are).

Finally, healthy fats are important for keeping your mind healthy and controlling your emotions. Healthy fats include nuts, nut butters, oils, avocado, and flaxseeds along with other varieties of seeds.

Never Shop Without a Grocery List

Grocery shopping without a list is potentially the most dangerous thing a binge eater could do, because items you shouldn't be buying will sneak into your cart. Just like when you start a new workout regimen and planning what you'll be doing every session at the gym, when you go grocery shopping you need to have a game plan to keep you on track.

Wandering the aisles aimlessly sets up you up for the fall. So writing out a grocery list before you go will prevent this from being a problem (this applies to your initial restocking now that you've tossed out the unhealthy food you shouldn't be eating, as well as in the future whenever you need to pick up food).

You should divide the list into categories such as produce, meat, whole grains, and dairy to keep your focus in one section at a time. Avoid the inner aisles as much as possible (for the binge eater they are the danger zones to avoid as they often contain snacks, candy and promotional items). You may have to periodically walk down them for things like natural peanut butter, flaxseed, oats, brown rice, and so on. But focus on quickly getting in and out to prevent temptation.

Going shopping while you're hungry can be the worst thing you can do, because you'll be subconsciously planning your binge and pick up problem foods to have on hand later on. Therefore, you should shop only when you've already eaten or don't feel hungry. You'll be far better off, and have more control over your food consumption.

So once again, never ever go shopping without a grocery list and stick to it!

Avoid Intense Diets

The next point that needs to be made is to avoid intense diets. If you're currently dealing with a weight problem because you've been binge eating for a long time, it may be tempting to go on a strict diet to get yourself down to a weight you're happy with.

But a radical diet plan won't work until you overcome your binging. Humans only have so much self-control, so if you're trying to overhaul your daily eating habits as well as the issues that cause you to binge, chances are you're not going to succeed with either of them.

If one area of your life is consuming your self-control, the less control you'll have dealing with other areas. For instance, if you're trying to avoid binging in the evenings, you don't want to have to fight against hunger as that's too much 'fighting back' for anyone to deal with. Plus, when you put yourself on a fat loss diet you're more likely to feel restricted (for some people, feeling like they're being denied food can bring about a binge, which is precisely what you don't want as that will lead you to trouble).

Instead, you should find a way to eat healthy but don't think of it as dieting. Focusing on eating enough so that you're satisfied will put you in tune with your body's natural hunger signals, which is what you want to avoid binging altogether. Avoiding any diet plan during your recovery will help you achieve a healthier relationship with food, and help you gain control over all your eating issues.

Toss Take-Out Menus

Many people satisfy their urge to binge with take-out food, so removing menus is definitely a smart plan as it's far too easy to order enough to feed several people when it's really just for you. You normally wouldn't go to a restaurant and eat three full-sized entrees, but with take-out that becomes possible.

In addition, most take-out places serve the type of food people love to binge on (pizza, burgers and fries, Chinese, pasta, etc), and now you have a real problem. When it's as easy as picking up a phone, ordering, and the food magically shows up, it's far easier to binge.

Stay Busy

When are you most likely to binge?

Many people come home after a stressful day at work, and curl up on the couch with good food and a favorite television show. Or they eat out of boredom. They also binge in the privacy of their home and away from prying eyes (some even do it in the parking lot at a fast food restaurant, so you'll want to stay away from there as well).

Look at your past behavior and think about when you were most likely to binge. Then figure out a solution to keep you busy and prevent the binge from occurring. For instance, staying away from the environment where you will overeat (kitchen, snacking while watching TV, talking on the phone) for just 30 to 60 minutes can side-step the binge.

Make plans to get out of the house – whether this means running errands, meeting a friend for coffee, going window shopping, or volunteering at a neighborhood crisis center.

Exercise releases feel-good endorphins (which can provide a similar result as if you had eaten a piece of chocolate cake). When you feel like you can't cope or are bored to tears – and feel a binge is on the horizon – treat yourself to a massage or a manicure, a walk in the park or a game of golf.

Anything that will relax you and get you out of the house. Chances are a brisk ten-minute walk will clear your head, work through some of the feelings you're dealing with, and you'll return home having averted a disaster.

You don't need to come up with an elaborate scheme to keep yourself away from home to avoid temptation – you just need to find ways to keep busy. Plan your schedule so there's less time to snack or binge. Everyone is unique in this regard, so you'll have to devise your own formula for success at thwarting a potential binge.

Eliminate Distractions

In today's busy world people seldom have time to sit down for a good meal. If you rush through the day and grab meals on the go, you'll come home feeling like you haven't eaten much and will grab what's handy.

Many people are in the habit of mindlessly eating their meals while watching television, surfing the Net, or reading. They focus on the distraction, and next thing they know their plate is clean and it barely registered that they had been eating. If this sounds familiar, it could be one of the reasons you're binge eating.

If you finish a meal unaware of having actually eaten the food – despite the fact you feel full – you won't feel emotionally satisfied and will head for seconds. You have trained your subconscious to eat beyond the point of physical hunger, which has gotten you into the habit of eating more. Second and third helpings will turn into a full-blown binge if you aren't careful.

But if you sit at the table with nothing but your plate in front of you and really focus on the enjoying the food you're eating, chances are slim you'll consume more food beyond that. You will have satisfied your emotional need, and won't have a craving for second and third helpings.

Do your best to carve out time at home and work to sit down and eat a good meal.

The time away will give you a mental break, and you'll be refreshed when you get back to your tasks.

Distractions while eating are never a good idea if you're trying to manage your physical and emotional hunger. Turn them all off during a meal, and you'll be making a good step in the right direction.

Eating Regularly Throughout the Day

For people who are trying to reduce their daily calorie intake in order to cope with overeating, or can see some weight loss taking place after gaining weight, skipping meals is a very likely occurrence.

You wake up in the morning and think that by foregoing breakfast you can 'bank' extra calories for later in the day. Mid-morning hits and you rely on coffee to get you through to lunch. When lunch arrives, you sit down to a small salad since you're watching your weight. At this point, you're still hungry so you reach for a donut or two and hope no one sees you eating them.

Then the guilt sets in, and you decide not to eat again until you get home from work. Halfway through the afternoon you experience blood sugar crash and feel weak and shaky, but hang in there until the end of the day. By the time you get home you're irritable and emotionally stressed from fighting off hunger pangs. So you head for the kitchen and binge on whatever is readily available.

If you've experienced this scenario, you need to take control and plan a smarter daily nutrition plan. This involves fueling your body at breakfast that contains protein, some high-fiber carbohydrates, and a small dose of healthy fat to get off to the right start. You'll breeze through the morning without noticing any feelings of hunger.

When lunchtime arrives, choose a lean source of protein such as chicken or turkey with vegetables and more healthy fats. Have a piece of fruit for dessert, then top your fuel tank off with a handful of nuts and a protein shake mid-afternoon. The difference in feeling like binging when you get home will be night and day.

Eating a balanced, healthy diet with weight control in mind doesn't have to mean skipping meals and being hungry for long periods of time. You may want to question any nutritional plan that makes you feel weak and shaky as it means your blood sugar level is tanking. The plan described above would be 100% acceptable for weight loss. But if you aren't looking to lose weight, you could add more carbs to your lunch and a mid-morning snack.

Taking time to get a good plan in place can mean the difference between continuing your binging or getting past it. Overcoming binge eating is looking at all factors that cause you to overeat, and your everyday diet is a major component.

Adopt a Healthy Exercise Program

Exercise is not only a smart thing to do for your overall health, it helps with the issues that cause you to binge. People who follow regular workout programs tend to be more mindful of their body, and are better able to stay in a healthy frame of mind. Focusing on an optimal exercise program can offset the desire to binge.

Exercise regulates blood glucose levels by increasing insulin sensitivity in the body. When blood sugar levels crash, people tend to turn to carbohydrates that supply the glucose needed to bring their levels back to a normal range. If the average person is more binge-likely when experiencing blood glucose lows, you can imagine what this does to someone who is at a high risk of binging because they deal with this condition on a regular basis already.

Exercise can suppress your appetite. As you put in effort at the gym and start seeing positive results, you'll get into the mindset that you don't want your hard work to go to waste. You'll take greater pride in your physical appearance, which will make you more mindful of what you're eating.

Keep in mind that a regular exercise program doesn't have to take place in the gym. While getting in a good strength training session is a very smart move, you can get your exercise wherever you can. This could be going rock climbing a few times a week, joining a dance class, yoga, or going for a nightly swim. Whatever gets you moving and improving your physical condition can reduce your tendencies to binge.

Eating a Lower Carb Diet

Eating a low-carb diet can be beneficial for a few different reasons. Like exercise, lower carb diets are far superior for controlling your hunger level. If hunger sets off a binge and you find yourself elbow deep in a bag of chips, you need to work on the source (what's causing your hunger) and not the outcome (eating the entire bag of chips). If you can find a better way to control your hunger, you won't feel the need to eat uncontrollably.

Carbs don't have to be junk food to set off a binge. A few slices of bread or a bowl of cereal may be enough to get you on the carb-train. You have a little and then you want more. Cereal turns into donuts, chocolate, and candy. So consider low-carb dieting as it offers many advantages from a weight loss point of view, and for people dealing with binge eating.

Additionally, if you're dealing with weight concerns due to previous binges, a low-carb diet will move the weight loss process along without having to count calories too intensively (which can be a trigger for some people, because feelings of restriction can lead to a binge). You'll sustain a reduced calorie intake you need for optimal progress.

There are generally two types of eaters. The first is satisfied with a small amount of food they're craving (which tends to be very common among non-binge eaters). They want a piece of chocolate, so they'll eat a small square and once it's finished they're happy.

These people do well with moderately adding treats into their diet plan, and don't do well on programs that cut out the foods they enjoy. But because they maintain self-control, they do far better on a program that has some flexibility for them to eat what they want in small quantities.

The second type of eater takes one bite and loses all self-control. A small slice of cake or a few potato chips just won't do. Once they have that first bite their desire for more grows, and before they know it the entire cake or bag of chips is gone. This characteristic is very common in binge eaters as they lack self-control, so it's best to omit the problem foods from their diet altogether.

So think for a moment about what type of person you are. Do you find it difficult to stop after just a few bites? If so, reducing many carbs from your plan (the types of food that tend to give most people trouble) will make it easier to stay on course and avoid a binge.

Meditation and Yoga

Another thing you can do to help you cope with binge eating is to become involved in meditation and yoga (if you aren't already). Although this doesn't at first seem like intense activity, don't overlook the power it can have on your mind/body awareness as it can help you tune into messages your body is sending you. (Part of binge eating has to do with being out of touch with your body and not being able to control the negative patterns you've established).

When you're in the middle of a binge, you certainly aren't thinking about how your body is feeling with all the food inside you. You're on a mission to fill a void and mask whatever pain you're experiencing by taking pleasure in food.

People with a very low mind-body connection stand a much lower chance of stopping a binge. Yoga and meditation teaches you how to become better in tune to your body and its needs, and learn how to take control of those moments when you have an urge to overeat. Granted, it will take work – especially when your emotions are running high. But with regular practice and commitment, a reconnection to a healthier mind and body is possible.

Many people find great personal growth through the meditation and yoga. So it's definitely worth trying if you're struggling to find an answer, as it will lead to many benefits in other areas of your life.

There is a degree of helplessness and shame that goes along with binge eating, so with these techniques you can learn that you aren't powerless and you can control your destiny.

Summary

You now have many key points to keep in mind regarding the physical elements of binge eating. The most important takeaway is that you must get problem foods out of your house and replace them with healthier options (which is perhaps the most powerful thing you can do to take control of your binging).

You need to work on the mental and emotional aspects of binge eating (which we'll be taking about next) in order to stop your negative eating tendencies for good, and unearth what's really driving you to eat.

So let's move forward and talk about the mental aspects of binge eating.

2. Psychological ASPECTS

Now that you know about the physical components, it's time to look at some of the psychological reasons behind your behavior. Many binge eaters justify their actions by telling themselves there's no reason to be concerned. But there's little chance to overcome your addiction until you admit you have a problem.

Positive Self-Statements

Many binge eaters are in denial about their situation, and won't accept reasons to stop even though they know what it's doing to their weight.

Poor body image can lead people to overeat. Although some people will go to one extreme and starve themselves literally to death, others go the opposite direction into obesity and self-deprecation. They aren't happy with the way they look, but don't believe there's anything they can do. Rather than find the motivation and courage to change, they simply accept the way they are. They're already overweight, so why does it matter if they continue to pack on the pounds?

Some people binge as a way of coping with their self-loathing for their body. Food is comforting, so they turn to it to escape their feelings. But then guilt sets in and they become even less happy about their appearance, and fall deeper into the abyss of depression and overeating.

A first step to overcoming binge eating is psychologically improving your body image. And one very good method is to practice positive affirmations. You'll want to begin by making a thorough list of all the things you do like about your body, which can involve the way it looks as well as how it feels and functions.

Perhaps you like that your legs are strong and powerful and allow you to easily participate in a sport you love. Or you like the way your arms have good muscle definition and feel confident wearing sleeveless shirts. Whatever the case, the main idea is you want to appreciate good things about your body.

If you have a negative body image, chances are you're always finding flaws. So the objective is to start shifting your thought patterns away from what you don't like to what you do like. By focusing on your positive attributes, you'll have a greater desire to stop your binge eating and regain control over your life.

Once you have your list of positive statements, read through them a minimum of once per day to keep them top of mind when negative self-talk starts sabotaging your efforts and heads you straight into a binge.

Strength Training

Another great way to enhance your self-image while gaining more respect for what your body can do is to start a strength training program. As you come to see just how strong and capable your body really is, you'll be more inclined to put forth the effort of beating binge eating.

First, strength training can help reduce your stress level by giving you the positive rush of endorphins you'd otherwise get from binging. A thorough program can increase your insulin sensitivity which helps ward off diabetes, and improve your cholesterol level which will help manage your risk of heart disease. It can also help prevent depression, which some binge eaters also experience.

Second, using a weight training program is a great way to escape when you feel a binge coming on. It was discussed earlier about going for a walk, but a workout session will work equally as well.

Finally, a strength training program will increase your lean muscle mass and improve your body's ability to burn calories even while at rest, which will help get you down to your goal weight. This means you'll have to diet less intensely, which will help reduce any feelings of restriction you may feel that can bring on a binge. In addition, many people find they get far better benefits from strength training than they would a cardio-based workout program.

If you're at the point where your self-confidence is so low that you aren't comfortable in a public gym, keep in mind that you can conduct a full training routine to perform in the comfort and privacy of your own home.

A total body strength training program takes around 30 minutes or so two to three times per week, so it's not much of a time investment considering all the benefits. If you have a busy schedule, wake up 20 minutes earlier to get your exercise in for the day. You only have to pick up a few dumbbells and you can easily work all the main muscle groups without any problem.

There's really no excuse for not starting a weight training program when you have the tools and resources to do so. This one simple addition to your week will offset many of the negative impacts that binge eating has on your health.

Recognizing Justifications

Another thing you need to address is any justification you're making for your binging.

Since overeating and obesity is rampant in today's society, it's easy to believe there isn't anything wrong with what you're doing. After all, eating massive portions in restaurants has become the norm. So you tell yourself that if other people are doing it, it should be fine for you as well.

But subconsciously you know this mindset is warped. Super-sizing meals may get you better value for your dollar, but it shows how little you value your health.

Many people like how cheap extra large serving sizes are (therefore more bang for their buck), or how little they have to pay for the larger size of snack food at the grocery store and justify this as saving money. It's especially enticing during BOGO (buy one get one free) or half-price days. Why turn down the second burger when it's "free"?

It's time to take a really good look at any self-justification. Whether you're denying the fact you have a problem or have a ton of excuses, until you can stop your self-sabotaging you can't expect to change.

If you're having trouble recognizing your justifications, the next time you sit down to eat more food than you know you should (and be honest about that), you need to stop and ask yourself the following questions:

• Why am I eating more than I need?

- Is it because the food is in front of me?
- Is it because others around me are eating that much?
- Is it because I have nothing better to do?
- Is it because it tastes good?
- Is it because I don't really care if I gain more weight?

Pose these questions to yourself to uncover why you binge. Once you've identified the why, then you can address the how. For example, if you see other people eating that much, you should ask yourself why is what they're doing considered normal? Then how can you ignore them and eat a well-balanced meal?

Start assessing yourself self-talk to see what justifications you're using. As you begin this journey into deeper awareness, you might be surprised at the negative messages you've been sending yourself for way too long.

Toss Fashion and Fitness Magazines

Another important thing you should be doing to get in a better mental place and improve your body image is to throw out all the fashion and fitness magazines.

Mass media marketing messages are a big reason why so many people have negative body issues. Flipping through pages of fitness magazines and looking with envy at the women or men that grace the covers or ads could be fueling your dissatisfaction with your body (don't forget that lots of airbrushing occurs before it goes to print, so an unrealistic, skewed image is used to sell the magazine). You end up feeling less confident and hopeless. You're too far gone for anything to make a difference, so you binge as a balm for your unhappiness.

Many media images are unrealistic for the average person to attain (many models and celebrities constantly starve themselves to look like that. Who wants to live a life of deprivation?) However, if that's what you view as an ideal body image, it's no wonder you feel helpless.

Instead, you should work on finding positive role models – people who are fit, healthy, and very self-confident. Watch how they behave and replicate this in your own life. A person with a positive self-image usually doesn't diet, but eats for enjoyment and the health benefits of food. Since they are comfortable with themselves, they don't obsess over things that can cause binging.

Eating is something they do naturally without too much thought. But this is usually not the case for the binge eater as they need to be in control of their eating 24/7 to stay in control. (A binge, however, provides the opportunity to loosen the reins and feel temporarily in control.)

Binge eaters versus "normal" eaters tend to have very different thought processes surrounding food and eating. So finding someone healthy to be a positive role model will be far better than trying to live up to unrealistic magazine images.

Eliminating Feelings of Helplessness

Many people feel helpless when they're binging. They've been doing it for so long that when the feeling that leads to a binge strikes, it's so overwhelming that it feels there's nothing they can do about it. If that's how you're feeling, it will be challenging to break free from any thoughts of despair. The good news is it's definitely possible as long as you stay focused and positive.

To help overcome your feelings of helplessness, you need to take baby steps to make sure you celebrate every victory. For example, when the feelings that lead to a binge strike, head out for a ten-minute walk to side-step them. Even if you do binge afterwards, it's important to acknowledge that you tried to avoid overeating.

Many people feel as though they're a complete failure, because despite their efforts they still binged. Acknowledging even the smallest accomplishments will build your self-esteem. So the next time you go for a walk and return you won't feel the need to binge.

Overcoming your feelings of helplessness means you're on your way to getting rid of the problem forever. The more you focus on the positive things you're doing while reducing the negative things, the less helpless you'll feel.

You'll slowly gain confidence in your ability to carry out a task, which at the end of the day is what will help you get over your problem. As your confidence grows, you'll eventually reach a point where you no longer feel helpless, and you'll feel empowered to carry out your goals.

Another helpful tool is to take a good look at what indicators are present when you're feeling helpless. One big error many people make is 'making a mountain out of a molehill.' They make one little mistake or have a setback and think they're completely powerless, and walk away feeling defeated.

The next time you're feeling even the slightest bit helpless, stop and take a good look at the situation. What factors are present that are leading you to believe you're helpless and can't get out of the situation? And what steps could you take to move forward? When you shift your thinking patterns, you'll see potential solutions and evidence that your feelings are justified, and that there are viable ways to manage the situation.

Most people are emotionally overwhelmed in the moments leading up to and after a binge, so these thought processes never cross their mind. You need to establish reminders to keep your focus sharp and your attention away from binging. For example, tape an affirmation or a photo of what you'd like to look like on the fridge or pantry door that will spark positive thoughts. A reminder can help you move through your feelings and correct them so they won't happen again.

Don't expect to completely eliminate those feelings in just a few days as it will take time to overcome them. Remember that you didn't develop binge eating overnight, so expecting to move past it in one day isn't realistic. But with the right frame of mind, you overcome it quickly and regain control over your eating habits and lifestyle.

The mind is a very powerful thing, and when it's struggling it's going to manifest many behavior traits that can and will cause problems such as binge eating. So don't be quick to assume that the issues you're struggling with are only about food.

This wraps up the discussion on the mental element of binge eating. Now we'll move forward and talk about another area that comes into play for individuals suffering from binge eating: Emotions, like the mental aspects, are very powerful, and must be controlled if you're going to move past binge eating forever.

3. Emotional
ASPECTS

Now that some of the main physical and mental aspects of dealing with binge eating have been covered, it's time to turn the focus to the emotional aspects that need to be addressed.

Many of the previous points will help you temporarily put a halt to binge eating, but they won't take care of the underlying cause since there's obviously something deeper than the fact that you like to eat. There are subliminal reasons why you start eating and are unable to stop until you're so full you feel like you'll explode.

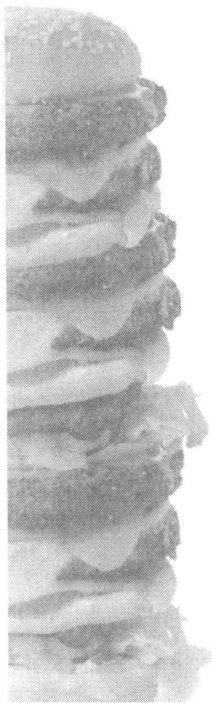

The goal here is to teach you how to deal with your emotional issues so that in time you won't have to worry about all the physical aspects, because the underlying drive to binge eat will no longer be a problem.

Journaling

The very first thing to be recommended is to journal your thoughts. Many people keep their feelings circulating in their mind and ruminate on them for days. So journaling is an excellent way to get your thoughts and feelings out – many of which you may not have known you had until you actually think about them and write them down.

There could be emotions you're not conscious of, and doing this exercise will help bring them to the surface. Then you can come up with a concrete game plan for how you will deal with your thoughts and feelings and get past them.

Set a timer for five minutes and write without stopping. If you can't think of anything to journal, write the last sentence you wrote over and over. Doing this will force your brain to reveal issues you hadn't given credence to.

You should do your journaling any time before a binge occurs (which is when your emotions are going to be at their highest). There's no question you will have emotional days, but not all of them may lead to a binge. Getting your emotions out on paper can help them from building, which could eventually lead to a binge.

While thinking about emotions can be constructive for working through your problems, sometimes it takes getting them out in the open. Writing things down is like expressing yourself to another person as the emotional release is the same. And journaling is a private, safe place where you can voice your concerns.

It's all about managing your emotions so that it never gets to the point where you're unable to control yourself. With practice, you'll start seeing the positive benefits journaling has.

Counseling

In some cases, you may not be able to solve all your issues on your own. The next step after you've begun journaling is to consider speaking with a counselor or behavior therapist. Dealing with very deep-rooted problems, feelings, and emotions is not something you can casually work through to find a solution.

Professional counseling can be of great help for many people, and is often is the only thing that will get them past emotional hurdles. You'll need to assess the nature of your emotions to determine whether they warrant therapy, and no one can tell you whether you need to go but you.

If you feel as though your emotions stem from childhood and you've been dealing with them for years, then chances are some outside help could be very beneficial. Likewise, if your emotions cause binging and other problems in your life, it might be a good idea to look into counseling. Of course there are many good self-help books and resources available, but for very severe issues they can't replace what counseling can offer.

If you don't feel you're dealing with serious concerns, then generalized therapy may fit the bill. But if you're battling other problems such as sexual abuse as a child, relationship trauma, eating disorders, or other serious body image problems, a specialized therapist can provide a higher level of help to your unique situation.

Having an objective point of view – whether from a therapist or someone you trust like a close friend – could be the very thing that helps you break through your issues. So take time to find a counselor you feel is the right fit for you. Being comfortable with the person you work with is critical in order to get at all the underlying issues causing your binging out in the open.

Find Passion in Activities

The next technique you should consider is finding activities you're passionate about.

One of the primary emotions that drives binge eating is boredom. You feel bored because you don't have anything scheduled for the day, or bored with life in general. Every day you're doing the same thing over and over, and there isn't a high level of mental stimulation that can bring enjoyment into your life, so you turn to food.

Food tastes good, it makes you feel good, and is always there when you need it. Feeling unfulfilled in certain areas of your life is what you need to be addressing. Until you're able to pinpoint what's missing and what causes your feelings of boredom, you won't be able to get past your binging tendencies. You will continue to eat to fill that void.

One of the best ways to figure out what might be missing is to think about what you enjoyed doing when you were younger. This may take you back to your childhood, high school or college days. Were you passionate about a particular team sport? Maybe you took great pride in working out, running, drawing, or playing an instrument. Think about anything you did where it felt like you were completely immersed and little else mattered.

This state of being is referred to as "flow," which is essentially a deep zone of concentration that takes 15 minutes or so to get into. But once you're in it you lose awareness of your surrounding environment and what you're engrossed in doing. Being in a state of flow can be very powerful for reducing stress, feeling greater satisfaction in life, and filling that void of boredom (which in turn prevents you from overeating).

So think of different activities where you would describe yourself as being in a state of flow. Then you should aim to perform them at least once a week and more if possible. If the activity is meaningful, when you're stressed and feeling emotions that would normally lead you to binge, you'll turn to this activity as it's your new mental and physical outlet for dealing with problems.

If you realize you aren't eating out of boredom but loneliness, you should look for more social activities. Many people fall into the trap of binging because they're not in a romantic relationship, or are tired of the dating scene. Expanding your social circle through new group activities can help you fill the void of loneliness, and you could potentially meet a potential partner.

But you might not have a social life or a new mate until you take the first step to find new activities that match what you love to do (i.e., you could run marathons and find like-minded people to associate with, or join a book club or a church association).

The key message here is that you need to identify the underlying emotions that are driving you to binge, and then get involved in an activity that will fill whatever void you're dealing with.

If you're journaling your self-assessments, you'll find a commonality in your binge eating that occurs time and time again. When you're able to identify this theme, you can tackle it immediately.

Visualizing

If you're feeling highly stressed or overwhelmed at work, or binging because you fear social situations and turn to food to replace the need for human connection, visualizations can help. This is a marvelous technique to show you the power the mind has to overcome adversities.

You can use visualizations in several different ways. The first is to help you gain confidence in coping with your emotions. For example, you're in a very high stress situation at work where you would normally feel overwhelmed. Your feelings build over the day, and then you come home and binge to release your stress.

Imagine yourself coping with that stressful situation with ease. You can see yourself dealing with it in a calm and collected manner (take note of how you feel throughout the entire process). Repeating this on a regular basis will give you greater confidence. You will have 'seen' yourself coping in a more productive manner, and will be able to cope that much better in the future which will prevent you from turning to binging.

Find Healthier Replacements

Finally, you need to find healthier replacements for an oncoming binge. This is similar to finding passion in other activities. But this point is directed more toward what you should be doing when a binge episode rears its ugly head.

Finding passion in activities is a preventative strategy. Finding healthier replacements is the reactive approach to help you bypass the binge.

For example, you might take a bath when you're feeling highly stressed and know that you're about to binge. Or you might call a friend and talk until the urge passes. As mentioned before, walking to divert the problem is a healthier alternative. Everyone has different needs and desires, so there's no cookie-cutter approach to this technique.

Think of five to ten different alternatives you can do the minute you feel you're about to binge. The list can be built on your interests and what you know will take your attention away from binging. The activity should take very little effort (no more than what it would take to go get food for your binge), and is something you can do to take your mind off food and control whatever emotions you're feeling. It's also a good idea to acknowledge those emotions and write them in your journal.

You might want to schedule different activities for different emotions. For example, when you're feeling highly stressed, you should do different activities than when you're feeling sad and lonely. When a particular activity becomes associated with an emotion, you'll be able to focus solely on what's driving you to binge.

If you're very stressed, you could crank up the volume on your favorite song and dance around the living room to blow off steam to get in a more positive mood and energize your body. Or when you're feeling down, a call to a friend may be a far superior approach.

Think about what kinds of activities you can associate with what emotions as you plan your list of activities. Then put that list where you'll see it regularly so it's always top-of-mind.

There are no right or wrong decisions as this is custom-tailored to your specifics needs. But the fact that you're taking a step toward averting a binge is a step in the right direction.

Now What?

You should never feel ashamed about being a binge eater as many people suffer from this condition. But it's only those people who can openly admit they have issues and need help who are going to move past it and become healthier.

But you must take control over your binging if you value your well-being. Letting it go on for too long can be devastating your ability to maintain a healthy body weight.

Sadly, binging is a condition often happens in silence. Many people carry on their overeating tendencies for years without anyone ever realizing there is an issue (or without them acknowledging they have a problem). When in reality they may be starving themselves during the day and binging at night, thereby consuming vast quantities of food and calories in the process.

Binging may start out as a problem with overeating. But given time – especially if high amounts of weight gain occur and the person is self-conscious about their appearance – the problem could escalate to a much more serious condition such as bulimia (binging and purging), and the devastating toll it can take on the body.

So it's very important to carefully assess your situation and look at why you're doing the things you're doing. And then develop proactive strategies to help overcome the problem.

Although this guide is providing you with plenty of options, don't think you have to do everything to eliminate your binge behavior. Some of these strategies may not be applicable to your particular situation. But as you read through them you'll see what resonates and combine several into a manageable program.

You know your body, your mind, and your situation. You've been given some powerful tools and ideas to help you cope, but now it's your job to put them into action. No one can take control of this condition except you. You have the power to consistently remind yourself what results you want and why you're taking action to stop binging.

Change is never easy, especially when it involves moving out of your comfort zone and breaking bad habits. Binge eaters tend to be introverted, so it may feel like a real challenge to talk to other people about what you're facing. But you'll be amazed at how supportive people are, and how willing they'll be to help you overcome your problem.

If you're still on the fence trying to decide if you do have what it takes to put this problem behind you, always remember your options.

- Are you happy at this stage in your life with your health and body image?

- Do you feel confident?

- What are you giving up to keep this binge eating going?

Really focus on the last one as it tends to draw a very emotional response out of most people. Think about all the things you could be doing if you weren't suffering from the problem. How would your life be different if you were binge-free? Focusing on that will get you moving forward in the right direction, regardless of how painful or scary it may be.

Change takes time and work, but you must try. When you reach a place where you're finally binge-free, confident in your body, and have control over the food you're eating, you'll wonder why you waited so long.

It's normal to expect setbacks and relapses from time-to-time as you recover from binge eating. No one is perfect, so to expect a smooth and bump-free recovery isn't practical. Besides, it's not the relapses that matter – it's how you deal with them.

Now you have several techniques you can start using immediately to get past binge eating. Hold your head high and keep looking to the future. You can't change the past, but you can change the future by taking action so that tomorrow is a little better than today.

Wishing you a healthy, speedy recovery!

EASY WEIGHT LOSS: SECRETS OF TAPPING THE POUNDS OFF WITH EFT

Health Research Staff

Contents

Introduction: Emotional Freedom Technique (EFT) **49**

1: What is EFT Tapping? 51

2: The Tapping Process... 53

3: Identify Your Eating Triggers.......................... 56

4: Creating Affirmations.. 57

5: Comfort Food is Not Comforting 65

6: Beat Your Cravings 67

7: Get Enough Sleep 70

8: Beat Depression.. 72

9: Beat Stress 74

10: Beat Anxiety 76

11: Dealing with Loss and Emptiness 78

12: Deal with Your Anger...................................... 80

13: Stop Making Limiting Excuses 82

14: Build Willpower.. 84

15: Think About the Future 86

16: Change Your Focus... 89

17: Self-Acceptance.. 91

18: Identify Negative Thoughts........................... 93

Conclusion **97**

Introduction:
Emotional Freedom Technique (EFT)

You're doing well on a diet, then something traumatic happens or you have a stressful day, and you find yourself turning to food for comfort. Invariably you don't choose a healthy salad or protein shake to get through your difficult time. Rather, you wolf down cookies, cake, potato chips, or any other food instead of confronting the problem that's causing you to overeat.

Everyone's been there. But some people have a hard time breaking out of the pattern of using food as a comfort cushion. The sugar and carbohydrates you consume during times of emotional duress have a drug-like effect on your brain, and make it difficult to stop.

When your relationship with food becomes dysfunctional, it's time to look beyond the 17-day, grapefruit, or low-carb diets, and look inside yourself. The techniques your friends use to successfully lose weight probably won't work for you, because they don't tackle the emotional factors that cause you to eat and subsequently fail every diet you try.

Of course losing weight can be challenging. But when you add stress, depression, anxiety, and other emotional factors to the mix, it can seem nothing short of impossible. When your emotions rule your eating choices, your mind will sabotage your body.

What's worse, being overweight and having a negative body image can lead to more stress and depression, thereby creating a vicious cycle with yo-yo and fad dieting that can cause more weight gain. Unless you address the underlying problems at the root of your unhealthy relationship with food, you'll stay on a merry-go-round that will spin out of control. But it is possible to break the seemingly endless cycle of stress, overeating, weight gain, and depression.

In order to win the battle of the bulge, you must wage war on the emotional problems that are keeping you from losing weight. Once you learn how to recognize, confront, and eliminate the emotional issues that can lead to overeating and keep you from living a healthy lifestyle, you can shed the pounds and live life as a healthy, happy individual.

Emotional Freedom Technique (EFT) weight loss is about freeing yourself from emotions that cripple your desire to lose weight. The process is simple to implement, yet advanced in its results and ability to address your problems from the inside out. If you have tried to lose weight and failed because you turned to food as a crutch in times of emotional duress, EFT weight loss is the solution to solve your unhealthy eating habits once and for all.

Everyone deserves to be happy with their lives and their body. Free yourself of negative thoughts and emotions that are keeping you from happiness, and shed the weight that perpetuates your unhappiness.

Attention All Eagle Eyes: We've had a number of people proof this book before we released it to you, but there is a chance you might spot something that was missed. If you find a typo or other obvious error please send it to us. And if you're the first one to report it, we'll send you a free gift! Send to: millwoodmedia@gmail.com

1: What is EFT Tapping?

EFT was pioneered in the 1990s by ordained minister, Gary Craig, to help people eliminate the negative energy that results from disruptions in the body's energy system. It's a liberating technique that can help you overcome fears, emotional problems, and the backlash of overeating.

Deepak Chopra, a mind-body healing pioneer, noted the "great healing benefits" of EFT; performer Michael Ball uses it to calm his anxiety before going on stage; cage fighter Alex Reid uses it to deal with the stress of celebrity; and pop star Lily Allen has used it for weight loss.

EFT tapping is a remarkably simple technique that offers profound benefits to both your emotional state and your weight. During the tapping process you place your fingertips in the same energy meridians that have been used in Eastern medicine (acupuncture) for thousands of years to restore balance to your mind and body. While you focus on a specific issue (emotional, physical, spiritual), you use positive affirmations and tapping to release negative energy, stress and thoughts to bring you into a calmer, healthier, more stress-free state.

In an interview with NBC News San Diego, George Pratt, Ph.D. explained that after tapping you are "then feeling relaxed, which opens up other ways of your brain working."

Although it may sound like New Age "hocus pocus," it's definitely a fundamental scientific process. MRIs have shown that EFT tapping has a profound effect on people's brain chemistry. In a study of 78 anxiety patients, 50% had a positive response to acupuncture using needles; whereas, 77.5% had a positive response using EFT tapping techniques. Brain mapping shows immediate and long-term results of increased normalization of thought, proving tapping is effective for immediate and sustained change.

EFT has a broad range of uses and is applicable to nearly every emotional and physical malady. Problems that have been cured or treated with tapping include chronic pain; anxiety; irrational fear; overeating; lack of confidence; depression; lack of self-worth; inner turmoil; claustrophobia; issues stemming from abuse; diabetes; asthma; anorexia and bulimia; high blood pressure; PTSD; dyslexia; and carpal tunnel syndrome.

Gary Craig (the creator of EFT) is often quoted as saying "Try EFT for everything!"

If you've been battling with weight issues created by underlying psychological and physiological problems, you have nothing to lose by trying EFT. It's free and simple enough to do on your own without therapy (meaning you can stop wasting your money on diet books and pills that fail to address the real source of your weight gain).

2: The Tapping Process

Before you begin tapping you should remove your glasses and watch as they can electromagnetically interfere with the energy.

Familiarize yourself with the points you'll be tapping (below) to make the process as seamless as possible. Pay particular attention to the points under your eyes, arms, and on your collarbone, which are less obvious and can slow down your tapping sessions. Eventually the process will become second nature, so don't be too hard on yourself if your first attempts aren't perfect.

Before you begin, tap what is called the "karate chop point," using the tips of your fingers to tap the outside of the opposite hand. Then you'll begin with the top of your head and work your way down through the points on your face, your chest, and finally your wrists (using your fingertips of both hands to balance the energy equally on both sides of your body).

- Tap the top of your head with your fingertips of both hands touching and curved (they should look like a lowercase "m") along the center of your hairline.

- Tap your eyebrows at the very beginning where your nose and brow bone connect (with your pinky and fourth finger), and above your eyebrows with the rest of your fingers (like an arch).

- Tap the bones bordering the outside corners of your eyes.

- Tap the area on the cheekbones that is about one inch under your eyes.

- With one hand, tap the area under your nose between the top of your upper lip and the bottom of your nose.

- With one hand, tap your chin halfway between the bottom of your lower lip and the bottom point of your chin.

- Locate what is known in acupuncture as K-27 (K for kidney), which is where your sternum, collarbone, and first rib meet. In order to locate it, start at the point where a man would knot a tie (the hollow), and then move both sets of fingertips down one inch. Then place each set of fingertips one inch to the left and right of that point, which is where you should tap your collarbone (in EFT tapping this is referred to as "the sore spot").

- Locate your next tapping point by starting with each set of fingertips in your armpit and travel four inches down under your arm (you'll look like a teapot with your arms out to the sides and your fingertips pointing into your sides).

- Tap the inside of each wrist with the other (forming an "X").

Traditional tapping uses the fingertips of your index and middle fingers, which have more meridian points than your finger pads (women with long nails may modify the process to use their finger pads).

Your taps should be solid. Tap each point for the length of one complete respiration cycle (inhaling/exhaling) which – depending on the speed of your tapping and lung capacity – will generally fall between five and seven taps on a single point.

Watching videos (or finding charts) about tapping can help you to locate some of the more elusive points and master the tapping technique. People tend to find the tapping process a bit awkward the first time they try it, so don't give up. Once you've worked from top to bottom a few times, your tapping will flow easily and naturally. Like most things in life, practice makes perfect!

3: Identify Your Eating Triggers

The first step toward solving any emotional issue or addiction is to identify the problem. Before you can create affirmations to address your unique triggers and weaknesses related to food, it's important to recognize the underlying causes that make you overeat.

Ask yourself what emotional issues you're trying to avoid. Whether it's the death of a parent, chronic stress, your marriage, or some other emotional issue, you have to find out why you're overeating in order to stop. Ask yourself if over-indulging in food has solved your problem in any way. The answer most likely will be no, it has not solved your problem nor will it in the future.

For some people the problem is buried so deep within their subconscious that they can't remember why they started overeating in the first place. For them it would be difficult to craft meaningful affirmations.

But for you, by using this guide you'll be able to create meaningful affirmations that will dig the problem (or problems) up by the roots. You'll learn to address your issues head on, rather than avoiding them by anesthetizing yourself with food.

Maybe you already know what the problems are (a divorce, your job is putting undue pressure on you, your kids are stressing you out), so it may be helpful to journal your thoughts and feelings. Write down how you feel when you eat, what you crave, and how you feel when a craving first hits you. Go back over your entries for the week (or an entire month) and see if patterns emerge. Do you start craving food when your spouse gets home, or when you boss piles more work on you?

If you still can't discern what is creating the negative emotions that cause you to overeat, it might be helpful to talk to a spouse, parent, sibling, or a trusted friend. If you worry about what may be revealed during your discussion (i.e., you talk to your spouse and it turns out your marriage is creating the stress, or it's something too personal to share), it may be wise to talk to an EFT practitioner (or therapist) who can help pinpoint triggers, or what caused you to bury your emotions with food.

Once you identify where your problems originated, you are on your way to tapping the weight off.

4: Creating Affirmations

Affirmations are considered the most important part of the EFT tapping process. Each person has their own reasons for emotional overeating, so every set of affirmations will be unique.

- The first step of the tapping process is to accept yourself.

- The second step is to open yourself up (often called "turn-around" or "allow" statements).

- The third step is to choose, decide, and step forward.

EFT practitioner, Karen Nauman, offers the best affirmations for each step of this process on her website (www. tapintoeft.com). Although they should address your own particular concerns, these are a pretty good place to start:

Accepting affirmations:

- *I acknowledge and accept all of me now, including the feelings I have.*

To begin letting go of the emotional guilt you're plagued with – or when you feel lost, helpless, or overwhelmed – you must accept that all your feelings are valid and they belong to you and you alone. You can't diminish their significance just because you think you shouldn't feel the way you do.

- *I am a good person.*

Whether or not you feel your weight makes you unlovable, you must accept that you're a good person in spite of your flaws. Everyone has things that bother them, and there is no such thing as perfection. Essentially it's your "flaws" that make you unique.

- ***I honor and appreciate myself for how challenging and difficult this has been.***

Being overweight can put a serious emotional toll on you. Give yourself kudos for having the strength to not allow it to break you.

- ***I deeply and completely accept that I am doing the best I can.***

Sometimes you have to accept that you're doing the best you can to overcome your weight problem. If you've been trying a fad diet, rather than addressing the problem at its root, you're fighting an impossible uphill battle.

- ***I love, accept, and appreciate all parts of who I am.***

Yes, you're trying to change being overweight. But until you accept the weight you gained and know you're doing your best to change it, you'll be plagued by depression and stress which will make it difficult to lose the weight. Once you are okay with yourself and accept all the beautiful things about you, you can stop the internal war you waged many years ago and start losing weight.

- *I thank, love, and respect myself.*

No matter how you feel about being overweight, you must thank yourself, love yourself, and respect yourself before you can begin to shed the pounds. Once you have done these three things, the rest will be easy.

Turning around and allowing affirmations:

- *There is a way.*

People who deal with chronic overeating and body image issues often feel hopeless. Believing there is hope is a big part of making the future you dream of a reality.

- *It feels possible that I can begin to put this behind me and let it go.*

If you've been beating yourself up over your weight problems, you need to let go of all of your feelings of guilt and worthlessness to open yourself up to new possibilities. Negative emotions lead to more stress, guilt, depression, and anxiety, and will feed your need to overeat (notice the word "need" as opposed to want or desire).

- *I will allow these changes to happen naturally. I realize I don't need to solve everything now, and can move through this at the perfect pace for me.*

Just because your friend lost 17 pounds in 17 days on a fad diet doesn't mean you need to. The ideal pace for sustained weight loss is one-and-a-half to three pounds per week. If you're averaging two pounds a week, you're well on your way to losing weight and keeping it off for life. Accept that you're not going to lose it all quickly as it took a long time to gain the weight, and it will take time to lose the weight. Putting a timeline on your weight loss will only burden you with stress and anxiety, and make it easy to become easily discouraged and possibly give up.

- *I'm open to finding different ways to look at this situation.*

If you've been looking at your weight gains and losses through guilt and anxiety tinted glasses, it's important to look at your weight loss program in a healthy new way that will encourage you, not discourage you.

- *I give my mind and body permission to help me work this out.*

Your mind and body have been at war for way too long. Allow them to finally be at peace with each other so they can help you work towards a solution, rather than holding you back from losing weight. If you conquer the issues that plague your life, your body will take note and respond accordingly.

• *I believe I can find peace with this new situation.*

Let go of guilt and shame. Be at peace with your new approach to life – one that deals with problems, rather than smothering them with food.

• *I'm open to more resourceful ways of looking at this situation.*

Using food to bury your emotions is anything but re-sourceful, so you need to open yourself to more resourceful ways of solving and dealing with problems. Look at them head on, knowing you can deal with anything and you don't need food to do it for you.

Choosing, deciding, and stepping forward affirmations:

• *I choose to relax, be confident, and be at peace at this very moment.*

Approach your decision to lose weight in a way that fit your needs. If going to the gym for ten minutes a day is what works, do it. Don't create more stress, anxiety, and guilt for yourself by trying to squeeze yourself into methods that won't work – you're just setting yourself up for the fall. You know your body and how it responds to stimuli, so have fun, relax, and be at peace with whatever exercise or food choices you make.

- ***I am letting go.***

In order to move forward, you must let go of any failed attempts to lose weight in the past and the issues that cause you to overeat. Once you let go of the conviction that you'll fail, you'll be on your way to a successful "body makeover."

- ***I am rewriting this family rule because it doesn't work for me.***

If you've felt as though it's impossible to lose weight because of your genetics (so you established a mindset that trying was pointless), it's important to realize that just because members of your family are overweight doesn't mean you have to be. Yes, genetics do play a partial role in being overweight; however, they are by no means the only factors. Throughout your life you're like a magnet pulling in all sorts of experiences, issues, and subliminal negative thoughts that you need to "demagnetize" in order to find your way back to a healthy body.

- ***I choose to be emotionally and physically healthy in a way that works for me.***

When emotions cause you to overeat, you shouldn't create unrealistic expectations, or try to adapt to a method that works for other people but won't fit your needs. You must love and accept you for who you are, including your unique needs for weight loss.

• *I will take it one day at a time.*

Make decisions that are emotionally and physically healthy for you today, then make those same decisions tomorrow. Eventually, those decisions will become a natural habit, and your long-term weight loss strategy will fall into place as it should.

• *I am reclaiming my personal power.*

If you've felt hopeless in your attempts to lose weight, starting again can be discouraging from the outset. Reclaim your personal power to give you the mindset you need to succeed.

• *I will be more open and accepting about this issue.*

Accept yourself for who you are. Accept your weight for what it is. Accept the emotions you need to deal with, and don't bury them with food.

• *I reclaim my sense of personal safety right here, right now.*

When it feels unsafe to deal with your emotions (but eating to mask them feels like the safest thing to do), create a feeling of safety for yourself. Explore your emotions with the help of people you trust and feel safe with, and without the crutch of food.

• *I choose to find new ways to work this out.*

If past weight loss attempts have failed, choose a new way to work out your unhealthy relationship with food, and address the issues that are keeping you from losing weight.

There are limitless empowering affirmations, so find what works and what doesn't. By crafting appropriate affirmations, you can tap out negative thoughts and emotions that keep you overweight, and tap into a more empowered version of yourself who's ready to lose weight and begin looking at life in a new way.

5: Comfort Food is Not Comforting

When you eat for emotional reasons, you return to the scene of the crime with certain kinds of comfort food. Sugars and carbohydrates have an almost drug-like effect on the brain, so as soon as you crash from the "high" you crave more, which adds up to a huge calorie surplus by the end of the day.

Just like a parent laughing at the naughty things their child does (negative reinforcement), sugar highs reinforce "naughty" eating habits for people who use food to comfort themselves during times of emotional distress.

It's important to realize that foods containing sugar and carbohydrates (which reduce to sugar) don't provide the comfort you're seeking. In fact, they exacerbate your problems by swirling you into a downward spiral of highs, crashes, and more weight gain, which elevates your depression, anxiety, and sense of worthlessness.

You may think of the foods you crave as "friends" (whenever everything goes wrong or you have problems with people, food is the one thing that's always there for you). But they are the ultimate "frenemy" that makes you feel better for a few moments but will sabotage your efforts in the long-run. And with friends like those, you don't need enemies.

Enabling a "frenemy" is forgetting your responsibility to your body image and self-worth. You'll feel being overweight is the price you're paying for whatever subliminal negative messages are in your subconscious. When you bury your emotions with food over a long period of time, you get further away from your true feelings and a healthy solution (especially when you can't remember why you started over-eating in the first place).

The longer you turn to comfort food, the more dysfunctional and difficult your problems will become. For example, parents who control their anger towards their children's misbehavior with comfort food not only pack on the pounds, they fail to develop good communication and allow those negative behaviors to persist. The longer their children misbehave, the more they become accustomed to pushing the boundaries of what is acceptable without any repercussions or punishment. When the parent finally decides to address the issue, the children will rebel even more than if the problem had been nipped in the bud.

Therefore, comfort food does not help you or the people in your life. It does nothing but destroy your communication skills, your awareness of your self-worth, and your ability to deal with your emotions. And dear friend, there is nothing comforting about that at all.

6: Beat Your Cravings

Even the strictest of dieters have their Achilles' heel food, whether it's chocolate, cookies, potato chips, or French fries. When you're trying to diet, your cravings seem stronger than ever which makes them nearly impossible to resist.

In order to overcome your cravings, you need to give yourself a little tough love and use EFT tapping techniques to rid yourself of the desire to eat unhealthy food. Australian energy therapist, Rod Sherwin, outlines the steps to tapping away your cravings that can be easily done at home and modified to suit your particular cravings.

- When you first feel a craving, evaluate how much you want that food on a scale of 0 to 10 (with 0 being no desire at all, and 10 being an intense desire). Put the food in front of you (i.e., cake) to do your evaluation.

- *Frame an "even though" affirmation. For example:*

  – Even though I badly crave this piece of cake, I deeply love, respect and accept myself.

- Even though I know this isn't healthy for me but feel I have earned it, I deeply love, respect and accept myself.

- Even though I would feel deprived if I don't eat this piece of cake, I deeply love and accept myself.

- **Tap your "karate chop point."**

- Work your way down your tapping points (refer back to the earlier section of tapping points) and repeat the affirmation during each respiration:

- Tap the top of your head with your fingers back-to-back on the center of your skull. This craving for cake.

- Tap your eyebrows at the very beginning of your eyebrows where your nose and your brow bone connect. This craving for cake.

- Tap the side of the eyes on the bones on the outside corners of your eyes. This craving for cake.

- Tap under your eyes on the part of the cheek-bone that's one inch below your eyes. This craving for cake.

- With one hand, tap under your nose by tapping on the area between the top of your upper lip and the bottom of your nose. This craving for cake.

– Again with one hand, tap your chin about half-way in between the bottom of your lower lip and the bottom point of your chin. This craving for cake.

– Locate your K-27, the point where your sternum, collarbone, and first rib meet. Tap your collarbone. This craving for cake.

– Tap under the arm four inches below your armpits. This craving for cake.

– Tap the inside of both wrists. This craving for cake.

• *Now revaluate your craving. Do you crave the food less or more? Has the craving disappeared?*

• Repeat the affirmation and tapping process until you no longer have a craving. Be patient as it may take several tries, especially when you're first conditioning yourself not to crave a particular food.

When you realize you're having a craving, just tap it away! Soon you won't have to go through the tapping ritual as you will have engrained a new attitude towards cravings in your subconscious, and you'll see them for what they really are: Your body's desire to anesthetize itself against emotional issues that need to be addressed to prevent further overeating and cravings.

7: Get Enough Sleep

One of the most critical components to losing weight is getting sufficient sleep. When you don't get enough sleep or the quality of your sleep is poor, it's easy to start packing on the pounds.

A study conducted by the National Heart Lung and Blood Institute revealed that people who only get five hours of sleep each night are more likely to be obese than people who get seven to eight hours of sleep.

Sleep deprivation can cause a host of problems by producing hormones that cause your blood sugar to become unstable, which can cause weight gain. For many people getting a good night of sleep is easier said than done, as they're plagued with too many thoughts and emotional issues to fall into a deep sleep. But EFT can be used to help you get sleep.

- Don't tell yourself to go to sleep as it will create resistance in your mind and prevent you from going to sleep.

- Focus on drifting off to sleep or being pleasantly drowsy.

- Use affirmations like "that driftingness", "drifting thoughts", "that drifting feeling." Or "Even though

I'm having trouble getting to sleep, I choose to feel pleasantly drowsy" as you work your way through your tapping points.

- If you're not able to sleep because an important decision is weighing heavily on your mind, try repeating "Even though I feel as though I must make a decision now, I choose to put all decisions on hold and let my thoughts drift." Or "Even though this situation is weighing heavily on my mind, I choose to allow my subconscious to work it out while I sleep peacefully."

- If you can't get to sleep because you aren't comfortable, tell yourself "Even though I can't get comfortable, I choose to enjoy moving and stretching while falling into a deep sleep."

- If you're fixating on the fact that you're not getting enough sleep, repeat an EFT statement like "Even though I'm worried that I won't get enough sleep, I choose to feel so relaxed and peaceful that it won't make a difference."

- If imagining your tapping points and utilizing affirmations doesn't work, try what's called the "touch and breathe" method, which involves lightly touching each tapping point and gently breathing while you think or softly whisper your affirmation.

Many people find they're unable to get to the last tapping point as they have fallen asleep. Once you're able to overcome your insomnia and get a full night of restful sleep, you'll be able to restore balance to your hormones and blood sugar, lower your stress and cortisol levels, and help your weight find its equilibrium.

8: Beat Depression

Depression is perhaps the most common emotional reason for overeating. And it can be incredibly difficult to lose weight when you feel as though food is providing you your only comfort as a salve for your emotions. Therefore, you must first emotionally free yourself of the depression that is crippling both you and your waistline. Once you accept that your feelings – whether positive or negative – are valid, you'll be able to cope with them rather than burying them with food.

Depression is difficult to erase as it's probably been with you for a very long time. So you shouldn't expect tapping to work immediately and will need to continue the process for many weeks (as mentioned before, your weight gain and emotions that caused it took a long time to develop, so it's unreasonable to expect overnight results). In order to overcome depression, you must first accept yourself (you can use the EFT tapping technique with an affirmation like

"Even though I have this feeling, I deeply and completely accept myself").

But depression may be too big of an issue for you to tackle on your own, and your triggers may be too deeply buried by years of hiding your emotions. If you don't know what feelings cause your desire to overeat, think about times when you crave unhealthy food the most. If you can't easily identify the trigger, journal the times when you're tempted to eat cookies, chocolate, chips, fries, cake, pizza, and other foods that are bad for you.

If you still struggle with depression, it may be necessary to seek the help of an EFT practitioner (or other professional) who can help you to explore, confront, and eliminate emotions that cause your temptations to overeat.

Whether or not you're able to beat depression on your own, if you have any hopes of losing weight and leading a normal healthy life it's critical that you recognize and accept your feelings. Once you own your emotions and realize you don't deserve a life of depression and anxiety, you can finally pull the problem up by its root and solve your weight issues (which no grapefruit, South Beach, or 17-day diet could ever hope to fix).

[IMPORTANT: If you are at the point where depression is seriously affecting important aspects of your life, or if you are considering suicide, please seek professional help right away. There are solutions for you to handle on your feelings.]

9: Beat Stress

Turning to food to calm stress is a familiar scenario for many emotional overeaters. It can be a difficult habit to break, as it's impossible to completely eliminate problems from your life. There will always be your boss, your job, your mother-in-law, your kids, the bills, or whatever it is that triggers your need to eat.

EFT is commonly referred to as the "ultimate stress management technique." While you can't completely eliminate emotional triggers from your life, you can learn to deal with stress in a healthier way that doesn't involve food.

You need to overcome your tendency to focus on the negative and start focusing on the positive with statements like "Even though maintaining a positive outlook is challenging for me, I accept who I am and how I am feeling." Or "Even though it's hard to be positive about the future, I deeply and completely accept myself."

First, work yourself through a tapping sequence that accepts your feelings about the present and the future with statements like "I find it hard to be positive about the future." Then work your way through your tapping points with a willingness and curiosity to explore other ways with statements like "I can shift away from these gloomy thoughts", or "I can become more positive", or "There is a different and better way to have positive thoughts."

Once you open yourself to the possibility of a new way of thinking, it's time to start focusing on your readiness to accept a new way of thinking. Use statements like "I am tired of feeling down" and "I want a positive change." Frame your statements about how you can focus on the present rather than worrying about the future, and how it's important for you to change your focus and maintain a positive outlook.

Now you're ready to start tapping into a positive, new way of thinking and looking at the world. Appreciate that you've worked very hard to change your thought process with statements like "I realize change can take a lot of time and effort"; "This will be surprisingly easy"; "When I become negative or depressed about the future, I'll shift my attention back to the present"; or "I appreciate that I am in charge of my thoughts."

By changing the way your brain processes stress you'll not only lose weight but the burdens you've been carrying around, and free yourself from the noose of unwanted negative emotions.

Everyone has stress, but allowing it to rule you can ruin your life. Learning how to enjoy the present rather than worrying about the future can help you to eliminate and deal with chronic stress.

10: Beat Anxiety

Although depression seems to get the most attention among healthcare professionals, many people face chronic anxiety that can be as equally crippling. Chronic anxiety can make you feel persistently anxious, and constant worrying can lead to a myriad of health problems including weight gain.

If you're the type of individual who turns to comfort food during times of stress and are on edge much of the time, anxiety might be at the root of your troubles. Anxiety is an inability to "calm yourself down"; therefore, indulging in comfort food is an easy, fast solution (although the effects will quickly wear off and you'll be back where you started, which begins the cycle all over again).

EFT tapping can be extremely helpful for sufferers of chronic anxiety. Even the physical act of the tapping can be a distraction from anxious feelings, as it keeps your mind off worries you're unable to shake.

Many people who find themselves overwhelmed by anxious feelings may attempt to fight past them only to have them unexpectedly crop up later. Utilizing affirmations can help you to accept that you are in fact experiencing anxiety. Understanding that anxiety is what you're currently dealing with, and acknowledging the emotions it can lead to, can be extremely useful during the process of eliminating your chronic anxiousness.

Begin your affirmations either silently or out loud, and work to accept your anxious feelings and acknowledge their presence in your life. If you can, try to understand where your anxiety stems from (i.e., "my relationship is unhappy" or "my daughter didn't call today") so you can identify the source and help to put it in proper perspective. If you can't find a source for your feelings, let the reason go and work through your affirmations until you feel relief.

I accept that I'm feeling anxious, and that is all right. Giving yourself the permission to have the feelings you're experiencing allows you to let go of a sense of urgency. If you're feeling anxious, trying to "fight past" your worries can considerably elevate your emotions.

When you begin tapping focus on the process, and don't allow thoughts to wander into your mind. If you start thinking about other things, bring your attention back to the sensation of tapping. It can also be helpful to count the number of times you're tapping, as counting can distract your thoughts. Other than your affirmations, a blank "slate-of-mind" is imperative to effective tapping.

As you work through the points, notice if your anxiety is decreasing. If so, pay special attention to the points where that started to happen and tap them again. You can repeat the entire process as many times as is necessary for your anxiety to dissipate. Once you've dealt with the anxious feelings, the urge to eat comfort food will be lessened, which in turn will help you to control your weight gain.

11: Dealing with Loss and Emptiness

Although food can't fill any kind of loss or emptiness (except the spare room you previously had in your clothes), many individuals repeatedly turn to eating when they feel despair or hopelessness.

Feelings of chronic emptiness can trigger emotional eating which can lead to a dangerous cycle of weight gain. The experience of loss – whether it's a friend, a job, or a spouse – can be overwhelming and emotionally devastating. Oftentimes, people can't figure out how to move past the emptiness loss creates, and as a result will turn to emotional overeating to replace whatever it is they no longer have.

The truth is no amount of food will fill the void left by something you've lost. Turning to food for comfort will only make you unhappier, which will lead to low self-esteem and further the cycle of overeating. Unlike anxiety, you don't want to allow yourself to just acknowledge the void; you want to fill it with something other than food.

EFT can help you to deal with loss and emptiness in the same way it treats other negative emotions. You can use tapping to relieve painful feelings instead of using food as a crutch or replacement. Tapping can calm your feelings, give you something to focus on, and use positive statements and affirmations to bring you back to yourself.

When you start tapping to assuage your despair, you need to identify your feelings using only positive language.

So the negative statement "I feel empty and alone" becomes the positive statement "Even though I feel empty, I have friends who love me and I am not alone."

People who have experienced loss or emptiness often become distracted from their current lives, and detach emotionally in order to stay in the past where they still had whatever it was they lost. This type of behavior can intensify feelings and lead to a vicious cycle of eating as a balm to their pain.

Therefore, you should use affirmations in the present tense such as I am not alone, or I surround myself with friends who love me. And focus on the positive aspect of the affirmations and your feelings of comfort during the tapping process. If a tapping point seems to respond more sensitively than others, pay special attention to it and continue to work with it until you feel relief.

Turning to food for comfort will only make your feelings worse, or shift one negative emotion to another. If you feel increasingly despondent, empty, or out of control, it can be helpful to talk to a professional. EFT can help you to get a handle on your emotions and identify them so that you're not tempted to eat to fill the emptiness.

12: Deal with Your Anger

If you're a "rage-aholic" and continually try to suppress your anger with food rather than lashing out, you can find yourself slipping into the "overweight" or "obese" category in no time. Anger comes out of the woodwork in many forms and for all types of reasons. Rage happens so often that society has come up with different words such as frustration, stress, resentment (and even "road rage"). The truth is that these negative feelings eventually boil down to anger (ergo, a person's "boiling point").

For women who are uncomfortable with angry emotions, this can be a particularly slippery slope sliding into weight gain. Society and their upbringing have implanted that it's not appropriate to express their anger (they're supposed to be "ladies"), and therefore must find another way to express their emotions. And for many that way is through food. Learning to recognize when you're using food to deal with anger is the first step towards changing your eating patterns and living a healthy lifestyle.

Tapping your way through anger is a slightly different process than, say, anxiety (with anxiety EFT you accept the emotion and work through it). When it comes to tapping your way out of your anger, you need to first deal with the emotions you're experiencing. Work through your taps for a few rounds, and talk through your heavy negative feelings as you tap each point. Let yourself fully understand your anger to identify what's causing it, and acknowledge how you feel about yourself when you become angry (this way you won't feel so inclined to "swallow" your feelings by overeating).

Do you feel disappointed or sad? Unlovable or out of control? If you don't feel good when you experience anger you can do all sorts of things to punish yourself, including overeating. Affirmations such as…

- *I don't like that I'm feeling angry.*

- *Anger occasionally lets me express myself in ways I otherwise would or could not.*

- *Being angry gives me a sense of power.*

…are examples of identifying your anger and the way it makes you feel. When you have tapped through a few rounds of thoroughly acknowledging your feelings, begin your tapping again and try to identify what triggered your anger. Was it a bad day at work? Was it your children? Recognize your triggers and use tapping to eliminate them.

If you utilize the EFT technique every time you feel angry, or notice yourself reaching for comfort food, you can get your weight under control very quickly. Anger is a natural emotion, and identifying it and working through it slowly is one of the best ways to handle it. Ideally, by the end of your tapping sequences and your acknowledgements and affirmations you'll feel calmer, less angry, and less likely to turn to food. In addition to tapping, you should learn other techniques to deal with your anger in a healthy, positive way. ***Anger Management: 21 Ways to go from Mad to Glad and Find Peace in Your Life*** can help you master your anger once and for all, and end the days of stuffing your face to quiet your rage.

13: Stop Making Limiting Excuses

People who are overweight often believe it's their destiny to be overweight. But nothing could be further from the truth. Everyone can lose weight once they overcome the stumbling blocks and excuses that limit them.

More often than not, stumbling blocks are horrifically skewed beliefs. You don't want to go to the gym because you're too big? Because you get sweaty easily? Because your clothing is uncomfortable and too tight? You're afraid people are watching and making fun of you?

Do you believe you'll never lose weight because of your genetics? Your metabolism? Your previous failed diets? Worse yet, are you afraid of succeeding at losing weight? Is it outside your comfort zone? Do you feel as though you don't deserve to lose weight? Did someone make disparaging remarks about your weight and you bought into them?

Once you realize that everyone, including you, deserves to lose weight and be successful, you can challenge the boundaries of your comfort zone and break out of the limiting thoughts that hold you back, and replace them with positive thoughts and affirmations.

Make a list of the excuses for why you're not working out or why you eat unhealthy foods. If you can't think of them off the top of your head, try journaling things such as the following for a week to see any patterns:

• Every time you come up with a reason not to go, write it down.

• Every time you eat a cookie or something unhealthy, write down why you felt you "deserved" it.

• Every time you think about preparing healthy food but decide not to, write down that reason.

From there you can craft EFT affirmations that will eliminate the excuses that hold you back from losing weight. Come up with a two-pronged statement: The first prong should include "even though," and the second prong should include "I choose."

For example, if you feel your genetics are keeping you from losing weight, you can use a statement like "Even though everyone in my family is overweight, I choose to rewrite this rule because it doesn't work for me." If you feel like you "earned" a cookie, create a statement like "Even though I feel I deserve this cookie, I choose not to eat it."

Most people who are overweight have a laundry list of excuses for why they're not eating healthy, why they aren't working out, and why they believe it's impossible to lose weight. These excuses will undermine your efforts, and by using them as a crutch will only become a self-fulfilling prophecy. Once you tap out your excuses, you'll realize the thoughts holding you back weren't as logical as you believed them to be, and were in fact toxic and self-sabotaging.

14: Build Willpower

Willpower is defined as "the strength of will to carry out one's decisions, wishes or plans." Taking control of your willpower is going to be the most important step to continuing the work you've already done, and help you stick with a healthy eating plan that works the best for you. It will keep you from reaching for comfort food during times of stress or unhappiness, since your "strength of will" will win out against temptation.

Many people who are working through this process wonder how they can build willpower, especially when they feel they don't have any. The truth is there is strength inside most people they never realized existed. And finding that strength and having the willpower to control your eating will help you immensely.

Visualization can be a good place to start building willpower, so think of your inner core as a tree. What kind of tree are you? What kind of tree would you like to be? Are you a graceful willow tree, one that bends but does not break? Are you a sturdy oak, one that stands tall and strong despite its surroundings? Do you have a sense of comfort that the tree (you) is going to be around for a long time?

It may sound silly, but this visualization can help you realize your inner strength in a familiar and comforting way. (Many people feel that trees are strong, sturdy, and were always there for them as children when they were swinging on rope swings, or climbing them with friends.) Remember the strength of your tree (the core of your willpower) when you have a hard time staying away from food.

Tapping is an extremely useful tool to building willpower. Create affirmations that include your inner strength, and focus on the tapping points that strengthen your willpower as you go through your session.

Eyebrow Point. One of the eyebrow point's strengths is willpower, as well as determination, restraint, and ambition. These are all elemental in building and maintaining the strength you need. Use affirmations like "I have made the decision to reclaim my willpower" or "I am discovering the strength inside of me and using it to build willpower."

Underarm Point. The underarm point focuses on willpower, your sense of achievement and satisfaction, your reasoning abilities, and your capacity for a clear thought process. Use affirmations like "I will build willpower one day at a time", "I believe in the willpower I have", or "My willpower is stronger than ever before."

Once you build your willpower to the strength you want it to be, you'll find that using healthier ways to deal with your underlying issues will become far easier. You might have moments of weakness and want to reach for food. But your willpower will remind you that you're stronger than you think, and turning away from unhealthy eating habits will become second nature.

15: Think About the Future

When realists assess the world they live in, it can seem a very unhappy place. Many things happen that they don't agree with or can't control. They may not be able to change their external influences and troubles, but they can change the way they think and react to them.

When people think about the future, many will emotionally respond to thoughts and situations with worry, stress, anxiety, or fear. All their negative emotions can lead to a midnight carbohydrate or sugar binge, and draw them back into an unhealthy eating cycle.

A healthy way to avoid this can be to define the emotions you have about the future, especially the ones you have about becoming a healthy eater, and deal with them accordingly. Accept that you may worry about what's up the road, but try to turn your worry into a positive outlet such as your creativity or an exercise program.

For example, visualizing your future as an unhealthy eater can prompt you to begin eating in a healthier way. Knowing that bad eating habits can lead to dangerous health complications can give you the kick you need to stay on track with both your EFT and your diet program.

Begin your EFT session with a "truth statement" (an example would be "It's sometimes difficult to keep a positive frame of mind about myself and my future"). Check how you feel about this on a scale of zero to ten (0 = untrue; 10 = true). Do you feel it's relatively untrue? Do you feel it's extremely true? Keep that number in the back of your mind as you begin your tapping cycle.

As you work through your taps, focus on and acknowledge the different emotions you have regarding the future that correspond with each point. At the eyebrow point – where the qualities of imbalance revolve around lack of confidence, fear of being overwhelmed, and nervousness – utilize a corresponding statement such as "I have difficulties knowing I'll be able to stick to my eating plan." Or "I'm tired of feeling nervous about my unhealthy relationship with food." This will help you acknowledge your emotions regarding the future of your health and eating habits, and deal with them accordingly.

At the end of this first sequence, go back and check your truth statement again. Does it feel more true? Less true? The same as before? Compare the numbers you determined on a scale of zero to ten, and remember where the feelings became stronger (if they did). Then give a little extra attention to those points as you tap through your next round.

When you work through your next round, try to use "turn-around" statements (sticking with the above example, use the eyebrow point again). An example turn-around statement might be, "I want to change these nervous feelings and turn them into something positive." Or "I'm certain I'll be able to stick to my eating plan." Do this throughout your tapping sequence. Check your truth statement again, and see where you are on a scale of zero to ten.

Finally, use the positivity and hopefulness of your affirmations to propel you into a future without poor eating habits. Use an eyebrow point affirmation like "Refraining from my unhealthy eating habits will be a challenge, but it's one I am ready to take on." Or "The future may make me feel tense, but I'm going to greet it with a positive outlook."

Worrying about the future is commonplace, as it's natural to feel a little apprehensive about the unknown. But with your acknowledgement of your emotions about your fears and expectations, you can feel more confident that things will be all right.

Your EFT sequences will help relieve anxiety or stress you may be feeling about your future as a healthy eater. And keep your mind on track so you can embrace the positive aspects of life, and no longer reach for food as a source of comfort to ease those feelings.

16: Change Your Focus

If you weren't busy focusing on food, what would you use that energy to focus on?

EFT therapist Ruth Stern, advises that "Anything you give attention to will become your truth." Would you get into sports? Spend more time with your family or friends? Pursue a hobby or career you've always wanted to try, but lacked the confidence?

Turning your thoughts around and making more positive and life-affirming choices can be difficult, but once you begin you'll find that it will become almost second nature. A good trick to start with is a follow-up statement.

Think about how much of your day is spent focusing on food. If you find yourself thinking about food in between mealtimes, follow it with something fun you'd like to do instead. For example, if you think "I've had such a stressful day – I want some cupcakes", turn your focus to something else such as "But that softball team is meeting tonight, so I should go to that instead." Or "I really want to call my sister and catch up with her."

Use your willpower to turn your thoughts away from food and towards goals you may have. In time, those pesky food thoughts will automatically be replaced with other things without trying.

Much of the focus of EFT is positivity, so it's naturally helpful for turning your thoughts away from things that make you unhappy, such as overeating, to things that can make you feel excited and hopeful. Several EFT tapping points can be very useful for you to help change your focus:

Thumb: This point can help you to achieve the positive outlook you're reaching for. When you find balance, a positive outlook about the things you want to do will come more naturally.

Index Finger: This point has similar balance qualities as the thumb. Both are excellent focal points for your positive affirmations about maintaining an optimistic outlook on your life.

Little Finger: The little finger point can help you maintain optimism and control your senses and thoughts, which will be helpful as you utilize your follow-up statements.

Collarbone: The "sore spot" can assist you in avoiding unwanted action. If you don't want to turn to food, focusing on this point can help you stay away from that negative solution.

Side of Eye: The side of the eye assists in inspirations behind decisions you make. If you decide to change your focus, you may find further information comes to you more easily when you pay special attention to this point.

Affirmations are incredibly important to the process of realigning your focus to a healthier mindset. You can go through your first EFT sequence and acknowledge each individual emotion that corresponds to the points. For the little finger point, you might use an affirmation like "I will be able to control my thoughts about food, and redirect them to a healthier outlet."

Much of the EFT process is individualized for certain situations, so working through points and affirmations is a very personal process. Determine where you would like your focus to be, and work your way up from there.

Utilize your EFT to help you visualize, realize, and live with a healthier focus. And soon your persistent thoughts about food will dissipate into thoughts about all the things you could be doing and enjoying, rather than spending time thinking about something that makes you unhappy.

17: Self-Acceptance

Self-acceptance can be the main turning point for a healthier and more positive future. Accepting the truth about yourself and the way you use food to feel better, calm anxiety, release anger, or deal with loss will open the door to change.

Of course you aren't perfect. You have flaws, faults, and things you probably wish were different about yourself. However, if you choose to accept yourself as you are, then any change you inspire will come from a positive place and will have far more positive results. If you try to alter your habits because you can't stop thinking negatively about who you are, the changes you make will never leave you satisfied.

And you'll want to keep changing the same things over and over because you never realistically examined them.

All your EFT affirmations focus on the goal of self-acceptance, especially the ones that deal with the most negative things like loss or depression. Affirmations like "I accept that I'm feeling anxious and I'm all right" embrace the feeling of anxiety rather than fighting it (which can lead to more anxiety if you lack the tools to combat it; then the change you tried to make probably resulted in more anxiety). However, utilizing and accepting your affirmations will make you feel calmer, more serene, and more in control of any anxious emotions.

Use your affirmations as often as you can. You can write them down and stick them on the bathroom mirror, and repeat them every time you look at your reflection. Affirmations are created by you, for you, and can be used by you any time you're feeling down or anxious.

Another positive aspect of EFT is the visualization technique. Many EFT practitioners advocate the silent tapping technique (the tapping you visualize in your head you don't have to physically perform). Silent tapping while you're lying down, or in the office when don't want your co-workers to see you tapping your face, can be very helpful in calming yourself down and working on your affirmations.

Self-acceptance can be difficult to achieve, especially if you have a pattern of negative thinking that's been pervasive for much of your life. You've tried diets and they haven't worked for you, and you naturally assume it's something you're doing wrong. Or you turn to food in times of stress, and end up having negative feelings for doing it.

These are the times when self-acceptance can come in handy, and utilizing your EFT sequences can make quite a bit of difference. Remember that change can come about, but it's up to you to make sure it's positive and not negative change. You can control the way you react to things and how you choose to deal with them. Accepting yourself as you are will bring you the peace of mind necessary to maximize the potential benefits of EFT tapping.

18: Identify Negative Thoughts

As you go through your tapping sequences, do you notice any surprising thoughts cropping up? These thoughts (or epiphanies) can give you insight into what's causing your eating difficulties.

Negative thoughts can be surprising, especially when they contain things completely unrelated to what you're thinking about. Try to pay attention to any negative thoughts and emotions, and if they keep coming to the surface try to examine them further.

For example, if you're going through your set-up statements and find yourself thinking about one particular thing, person, or event, give that thought attention as it's a red flag. Triggers that cause you to turn to food can come in forms you least expect, so you'll need to spend time on those negative emotions.

If you find yourself regularly swimming in negative thoughts (especially when you're trying to do positive work on yourself), try a sequence that solely addresses the negativity. You'll need a truth statement, a set-up statement, and a sequence statement (and remember to custom-tailor the process to your particular situation).

Create a truth statement such as "It's impossible for me to be a positive person," then rate that statement on a scale of zero to ten. Where are you? Where would you like to be? What kinds of negative thoughts do you have that prevent you from being positive?

Your set-up statements can deal with self-acceptance and forgiveness. On your K-27 point use a set-up statement like "Even though I may lean toward negativity, I accept and love myself just the way I am." Acceptance can go a long way towards helping you to feel better about yourself and resolve what is troubling you.

Tap through your first sequence and examine your negative thoughts during the process. When you have completed this, check your truth statement. Is it more true? Less true? The same as it was before?

Begin another tapping sequence. While tapping on your K-27 point, give a slight variation on your previous set-up statement such as "Although I accept my negative side, I am open to changing the way I think." Or "I accept myself as I am, but I don't want to continue getting down on myself for it." Let your new statements provide the basis for this turn-around sequence.

Work through your points again, but this time do the same utilizing your earlier tapping statements. Twist them around or re-word them so that each negative thought has a positive outcome. For example, "I am ready to let myself move past these negative thoughts." Or "I am choosing to look at life from the bright side from now on."

On your third sequence, allow yourself to think positive-ly. Focus on the future, your new resolve to think positively, and your openness to accepting yourself and your faults.

Paying attention to negative thoughts may seem coun-ter-intuitive, but in the long run can lead you to the root of your triggers. Turning them around will help you to move through this phase, and come out the other side as a more positive, much better person emotionally and physically.

If you've been using food to deal with negativity, chang-ing your outlook will help you stay committed to a healthier and happier lifestyle.

Conclusion

Losing weight can be hard for most people. If you've been using food to avoid your emotions, the process becomes even harder. Making real, positive, lasting changes to your eating habits, and your techniques for dealing with your emotions and your weight, will undoubtedly be one of the most arduous trials you will ever face.

It's easy to turn to carbohydrates and sugar that produce a drug-like effect. But it's difficult to think and behave in new ways. Although you will face difficulty and hurdles, once you realize what your life could be like without being overweight, avoiding your emotions, constantly thinking about food, or hating yourself and your body, it will be well worth the effort.

EFT tapping can be an extremely useful technique to help you through your difficult journey, as it's an incredibly empowering process to regaining control of your emotions, and learning to love and accepting yourself for the person you are. It helps you acknowledge your feelings, replace negative thought and eating patterns with positive ones, and gives you rewards for the hard work you're doing to put your emotions and weight on the right path.

Sometimes you may need a helping hand to keep you from veering off the path you've chosen to take. If you have trouble getting the hang of the tapping process and formulating affirmations unique to your situation and emotions (and how to get them to work for you), it may be helpful to see an EFT practitioner a few times.

Eventually the process of tapping will become second nature to you, whether you're providing the physical taps you need to ingrain the process in your mind, working through your tapping process silently at work, or when calming yourself down to sleep.

It's time to start walking without emotional crutches and living the life you're meant to live as a healthy, emotionally balanced individual. By tapping your way to successful weight loss, you'll find a successful outcome to your goals is much closer than you ever could have imagined.

Healthy journey!

Urgent Plea!

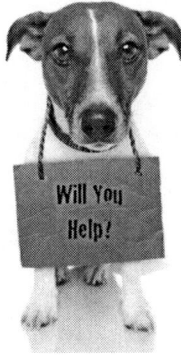

Thank you for downloading my bosses' book! It will really help life around here. Would you please help our Health Research Staff (and me) and go back to the site where you purchased this book and leave your feedback. They need your feedback to make the next version better. Arf! Arf!

CPSIA information can be obtained at www.ICGtesting.com
Printed in the USA
LVOW101618190613

339339LV00017B/666/P